WHY AM I SCARED OF EVERYTHING?

A Diary of Our Greatest Worries and Inspirational Quotes to Remember

BETHANY STRAKER

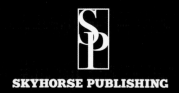

SKYHORSE PUBLISHING

WHY AM I
SCARED OF
EVERYTHING?

Inspirational Thoughts and Terrifying Fears...

the Musings of Regina Sharpe, Age 29

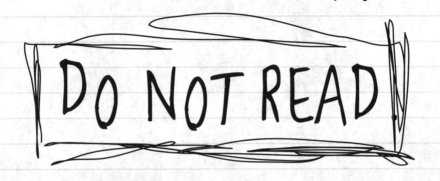

DO NOT READ

(Mom, if that's you, back away.
I am sorry for worrying you, though.
I always worry I'm worrying you all the time.
But if you're reading this, you might
have good reason to worry.)

Death

I have a little fear of death. It doesn't take over my life exactly
. . . but maybe I could do without stalking my doctor to ask
him if that lump on my head is a normal lump or a death lump.
Yesterday, I saw him run into a women's hairdressers in some kind
of panic. Probably because he'd seen me.

Woke up this morning and couldn't feel my arms. Tried desperately
to roll out of bed and Google my symptoms, and luckily the feeling
came back in the form of pins and needles, so I lived for another
few hours, at least. Not my ideal start to the day. Getting up in
the morning is pretty terrifying in general.

Then I made myself some coffee, which is now making
my heart beat too fast. Unless it's a heart attack.
And I have this weird ringing in my ears, which may or may not
mean imminent death.

Avoiding death is easier if you stay at home. But if I'm left alone
for too long, I'll have an embarrassing, improbable accident that will
be photographed after my death and put up on the Internet. . . .

CHARGER! Where is it? If I don't keep my phone charged, I can't call
anyone to tell them I'm dying. . . .

"Dream as if you'll live forever. Live as if you'll die today."

CR JAMES DEAN ଚ

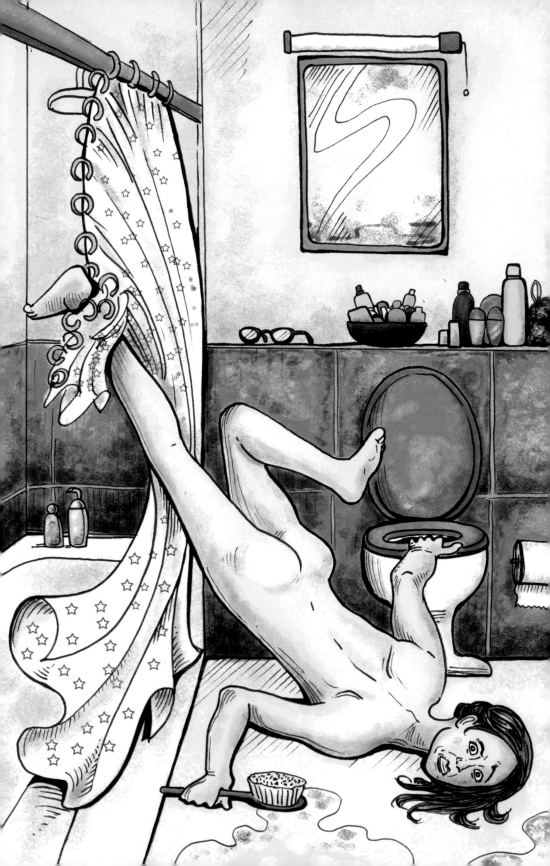

Aging

Just returned from the department store with my friend Claire, full of mirrors lit by Satan. My eyes have developed dark circles. When I smile my entire face creases up. Not just my eyes, but MY WHOLE FACE. This is the future: a long, downhill slide into ugliness and awfulness. People will be repelled by my face. I will never see happiness again.

Why is it that everyone on TV is twenty-one? Or fifteen? They all dance around in little shorts and look disgusted by people in their mid-twenties. Is this what's happening now?

My neck is getting shorter. It's getting shorter and it's framed by the flappy jowls on my face. The dress Claire made me buy is making me look like a character from The Others. Remember that part when the child turns around and has the face of an old hag? Me. She told me it was flattering! Right. It's going back.

"Beauty is all very well at first sight; but who ever looks at it when it has been in the house three days?"

ᘓ GEORGE BERNARD SHAW ᘔ

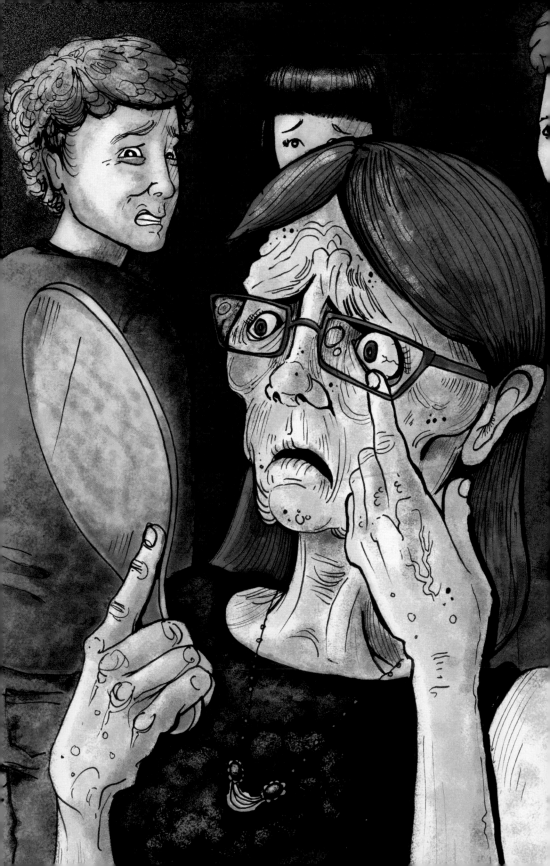

Credit card debt

I don't know what's going on with my bank. Did I check my statement? When did I check it? I think my bank thinks I'm dead, and when they find out I've spent all this money, they'll cut me off.

I had a missed call from a weird number today. Was that missed call from the bank telling me I owe them my car?

Oh my god, I have a lot of shoes and coats.

I also have a lot of cheese. I don't know why I buy so much cheese.

I've never actually used that foot spa I bought.

Maybe I can fix the hole in the roof myself? And the heating? Looks straightforward. In the meantime, I can just wrap myself up in all these sweaters I bought!

"A bank is a place that will lend you money if you can prove that you don't need it."

BOB HOPE

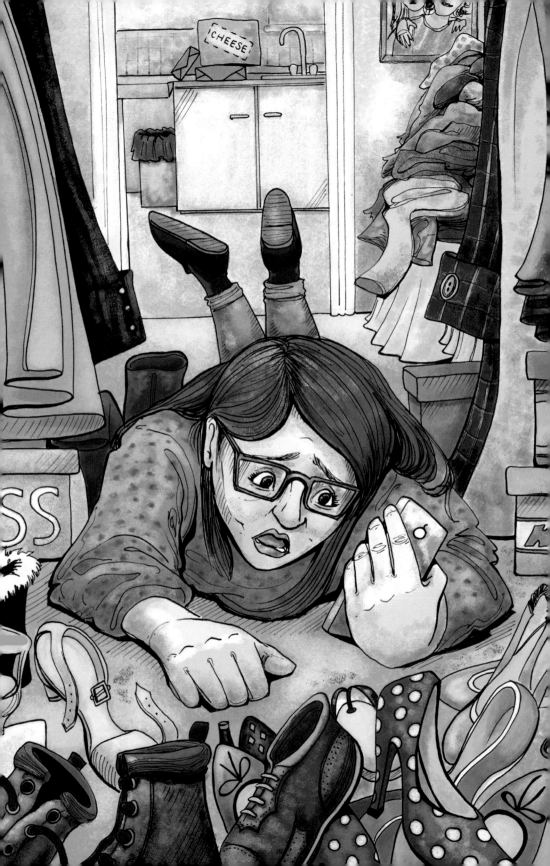

Environment

I was trying to eat my diet low-carb low-sugar low-joy cereal this morning, but the news was ruining it. They were telling me it's basically only a matter of time before we are all wiped out and I either die or have to select some animals to put on a boat. And then what if I can't find two of every animal?

Leonardo DiCaprio keeps telling me on Twitter about a lot of imminent disasters and things I need to do to save the world. So, I must donate some of my cheese fund to help the planet. I am feeling slightly less anxious at the thought of this, so I am going to watch a nice movie and go to bed.

GOD. If you don't want to worry about the planet, DO NOT watch a disaster movie. I have just emptied my cheese fund into all the green charities I could think of and called Claire. She told me I need to remember that there are people more experienced than John Cusack to help out the planet and that we probably have a few more years left in us yet.

Peppermint tea.

"It's not that easy being green."

ℂℜ JOE RAPOSO ℬⱯ

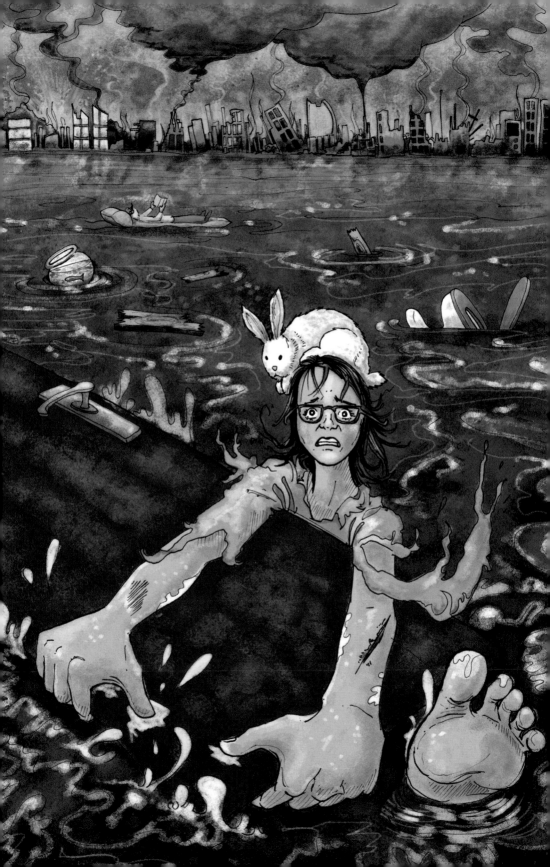

Failure

Coffee with Claire can lead to "advice" I don't want. "You're unhappy in your job, Regina. You need a new career, Regina." If I stop being a graphic designer, I will be broke my entire life. I will fail, and I will never be taken seriously, and I won't be able to afford to feed my cat. Perhaps the cat will end up eating me.

Claire thinks I need a five-year plan. I'm not Stalin; I can't come up with a five-year plan. I can just about think up a five-day plan, as long as it involves red wine at the end of most of those days.

Changing my job means changing my identity. Oh god. My identity is currently pretty non-identifiable, then.

"Ever tried. Ever failed. No matter. Try again.
Fail again. Fail better."

CR SAMUEL BECKETT ꝶ

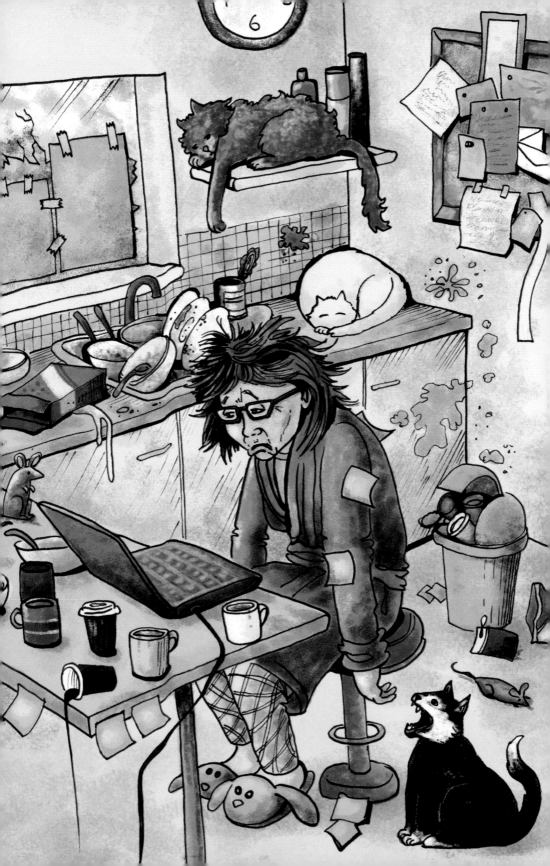

Friendship

I sent a group email around to my friends about some drinks last night. Not one reply. They're busy. I mean, we are all so busy, aren't we?

Okay, it's been another hour, and they've all gone into work. They're all at their desks. They're all deliberately not replying to my email. They're all probably meeting up anyway. Without me.

I knew they didn't like me. It's because I don't hug them like a normal person. But that's not my fault. I'm from a weird family of non-huggers.

Claire will reply. She is the one I can rely on. I'll just wait for Claire to reply. Then I will know she likes me.

"The only reward of virtue is virtue,
the only way to have a friend is to be one."

CR RALPH WALDO EMERSON ℬ

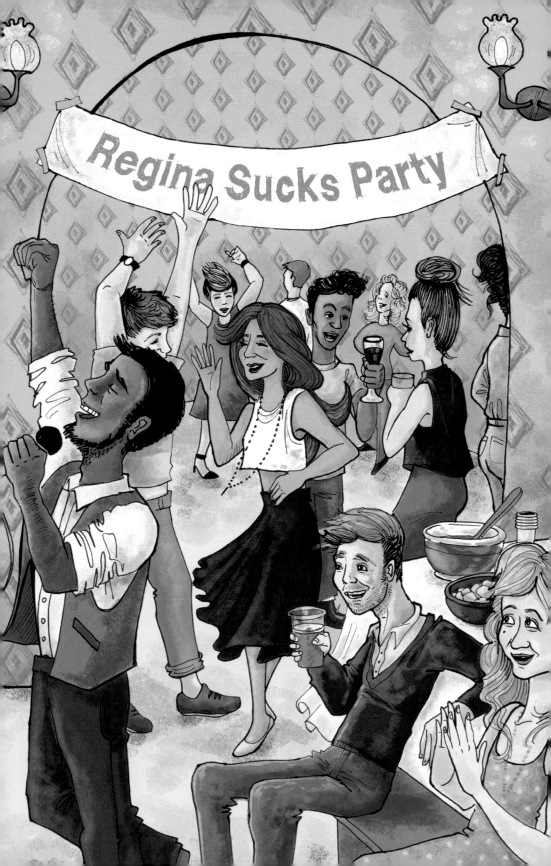

Embarrassment

I was having a bottle of red wine (I didn't finish ALL of it), and a pizza, and some chocolate and potato chips and a small gin and tonic and a bowl of fries. I might have spilled a lot of it on my white floral pajamas. I was watching America's Next Top Model. Season 84, or something. Then my stupid hot neighbor knocks on the door and I answer it in the middle of Tyra Banks shouting at a poor pretty person, with food in my teeth and my hair in a "comedy" updo.

When I leave the house, I am always unable to walk in my chosen shoes. When I talk to strangers, I accidentally spit. When people ask me for directions, I barely know where I am, let alone where they're going.

I'm pretty sure most people are stifling a laugh when they look at me.

"No one can make you feel inferior without your consent."

ᨒ ELEANOR ROOSEVELT ᨒ

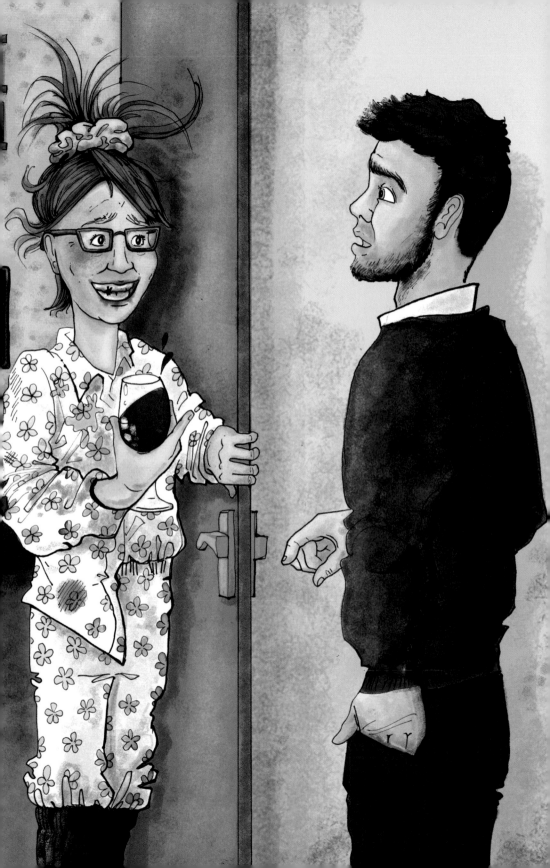

Flying

Home after a car sprayed a lake of rainwater into my face and thinking about getting away from it all. But flying? Does anyone else realize that if we all get onto a plane with so many people in a small space, statistically that must mean there's a bomber on board? I don't need to do any research.

The other thing to consider during a flight is that while we are all cheerfully eating our reheated chicken bits, we are sitting in a giant metal tube in the sky. IN THE SKY. Sitting in the sky. And everyone is having a nice conversation about their holidays.

Have we all just lost our minds? How is this working? Oh, right, yeah. PHYSICS. And the pilot falling asleep and the birds flying into the engines and something catching fire is all just fine, too. Luckily, they all just really put you at ease in these places, don't they?

"Just walk through this machine and we'll look at you naked, ma'am, and then we'll glare at you."

"Stay in the line please, ma'am. We all have to make sure you're in a bad enough mood by the time you board the plane."

I'm getting a train to the coast.

"Both optimists and pessimists contribute to our society. The optimist invents the airplane and the pessimist the parachute."

GIL STERN

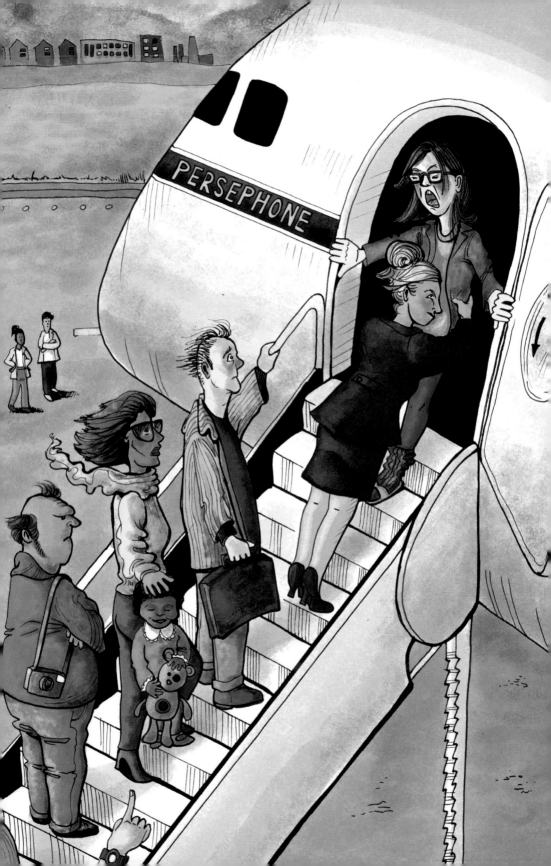

Relying on my Parents

Today I had the most excruciating lunch with Mom and Dad. Sitting in this wonderful restaurant, eating the most delicious food, my parents paying for everything. Right before I ask them for financial help. Dad just immediately said, "Of course! We know you're struggling a bit at the moment."

Oh god. Struggling.

Mom followed with, "Would it help if you moved back in?"

I don't think they thought they'd hit the jackpot when I grew up. Not exactly a case of their daughter smashing that glass ceiling like a pro and taking home a huge paycheck every month. It may have been a dream my mom must have had once, until she probably woke up and screamed with the realization that her daughter is a failure.

I am going to use a small portion of their money for a medicinal glass of wine to help me think of ways to make huge amounts of cash.

"In time of test, family is best."

ᘓ BURMESE PROVERB ᘔ

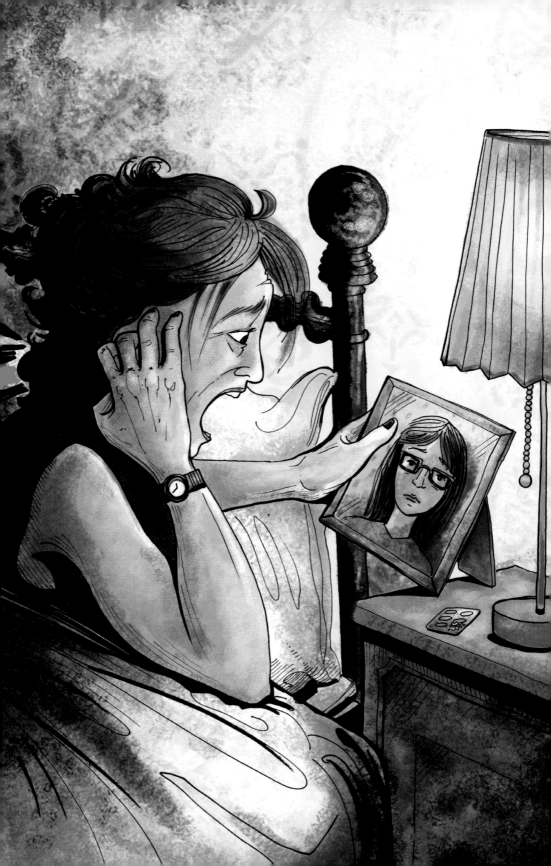

Becoming a Bag Lady

I was up all night thinking about my parents' offer to move back home. I shuffled to the kitchen and opened the depleted fridge, staring at it for a few minutes, flitting between what it would mean if I stayed living here and why I was still refusing to throw out that antique jar of hummus.

The rent is just too much now. I can't stay. I can just about afford a shopping cart, so maybe if I wore all my clothes and wheeled around the rest of my things, I could become a bag lady. I'll find another nice bag lady to hang out with, and we can sit on the sidewalk together playing Connect Four.

Maybe after a while we'll start following people around, just to mutter at them when they least expect it. We'll have some fun suddenly shouting out and frightening people. It will be a small glimmer of light in my new life.

I'll start collecting unnecessary things, too, to impress Sandy with. Sandy is my bag lady friend. We'll swap pieces of cardboard and give each other gifts of foil that we'll make into sculptures.

I realized I was spending money keeping the fridge door open, so I slammed it shut and crawled back into bed.

"Empty pockets never held anyone back.
Only empty heads and empty hearts can do that."

NORMAN VINCENT PEALE

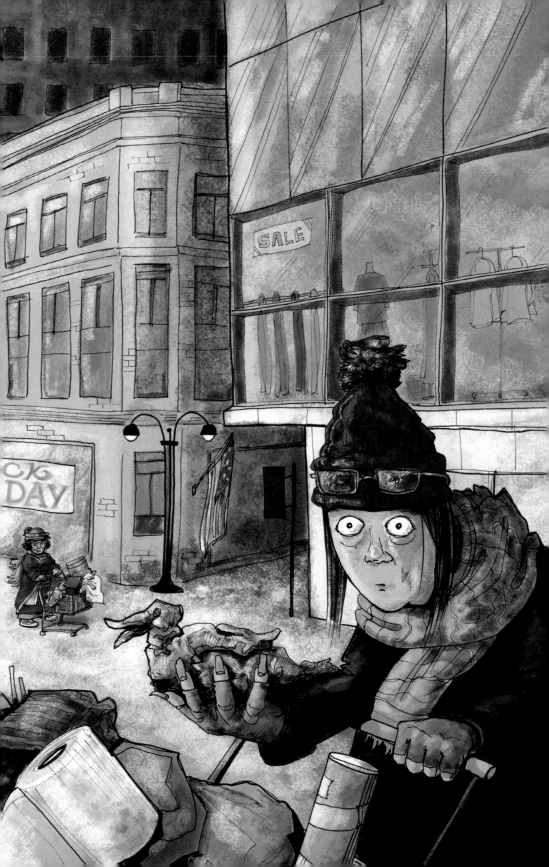

Property

Terrible, AWFUL news. Claire is buying an apartment.

I told her I was pleased for her, obviously. I am pleased for all my other friends in their lovely little homes they have bought for themselves, too. I do not in any way feel pressured to do the same.

Except that I do. Horribly, stiflingly pressured. I thought we were all in the same boat. I thought we all walked past those windows with all those expensive properties and said to ourselves, "Yeah, right!"

But all along, Claire has been the one behind the window, talking to the realtor, smiling happily at the thought of owning her own place. All those times I had bought my fifth glass of wine, Claire had saved her money for the Sensible Fund. Wasn't it just a few years ago we were all in college? The biggest thing I bought then was a guitar. That was a huge commitment. And now we have commitment coming out of our ears.

Eating a cold take-out pizza and guzzling a beer.
Not feeling too grown up.

"Any old place I can hang my hat is home sweet home to me."

ℭ℞ WILLIAM JEROME ℬ

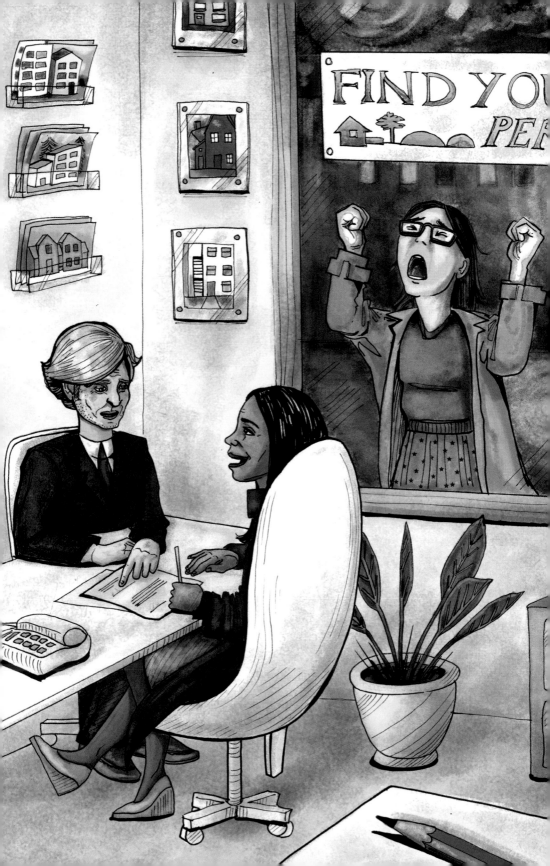

Weight

Oh, NO, NO, NO! That pizza was a bad idea. What was I thinking? And the wine, potato chips, and chocolate mousse? I woke up with this feeling of dread and darkness. I always do after a binge night. But today my chest got all tight and I had an urge to weigh myself.

I never weigh myself. Never—unless I've had a really, really bad month. Ideally, people should only weigh themselves after a healthy spell, but I only weigh myself when I know the results are going to be bad. And this morning they were bad.

Of course, after that I felt it was best to put on my tightest jeans to see if they still fit. They do. It's just I look like I'm wearing two blue condoms and a rubber ring.

As further punishment, I elected to wear this outfit all day as a reminder of my sins. It helped me say no to the donuts passed around at work. It did not help me say no to the double portion of pasta carbonara for dinner, but by then I had changed into my pajamas.

Peppermint tea.

"Use, do not abuse. . . .
Neither abstinence nor excess ever renders man happy."

ᑕᏰ VOLTAIRE ᏰᏜ

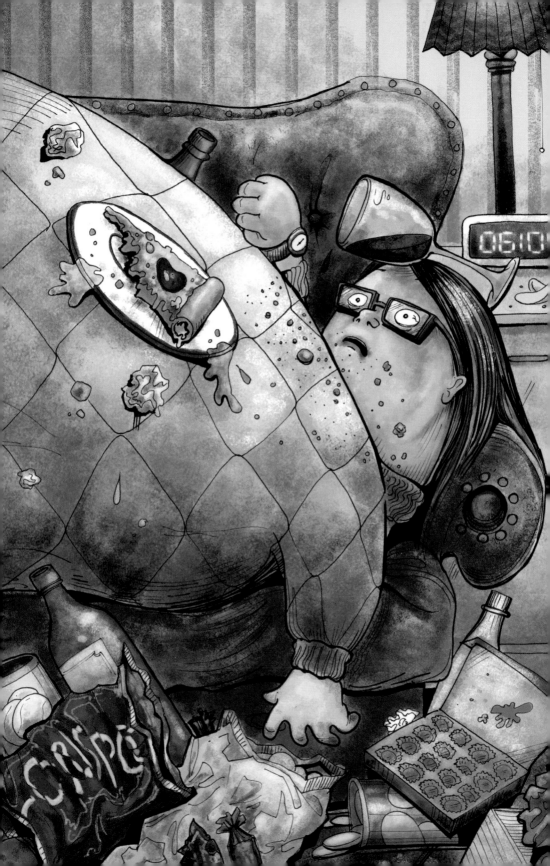

Bumping into an Ex

I went with Claire to help her buy some stuff for her new place. She told me about a store that sells those fashionable beaten up things that look like office filing cabinets after an earthquake.

When we got out of the car, I realized. I'M IN THE SAME TOWN MY EX LIVES IN. So that ruined the entire trip. I kept ferociously beaming at Claire, just grinning at her maniacally, tossing my hair around and keeping my stomach held in. She had to actually stop me to ask if I was having some kind of attack. If my ex saw me, he would have to see me AT MY BEST. I was even considering buying myself a cocktail dress to change into.

Claire is not usually one to put up with this kind of stuff, but she saw how pathetic I was and didn't hang around. She bought the filing cabinet thing and we skidded out of town like Thelma and Louise.

"Other people's opinion of you does not have to become your reality."

CR LES BROWN 80

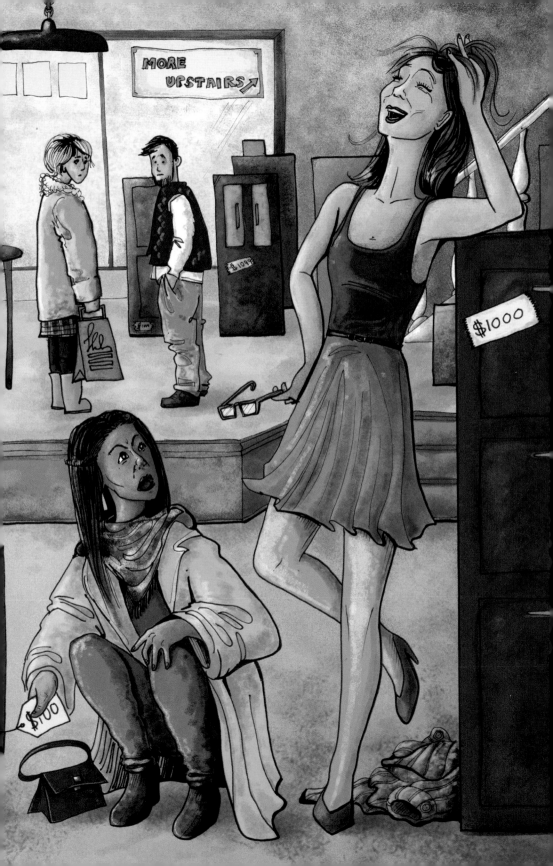

Terrorism

I'm on the subway and someone ACTUALLY HAS A BOMB because they are carrying a bag onto public transit and they're not making eye contact with anyone. I have to get off on the next stop. Should I warn people? That woman seems to know about it. But there's something in her expression . . . she has a bomb, too! She has an actual bomb. This is the end. Okay, so it's her baby. I need to get off and breathe in a paper bag.

I have gotten off in a weird station. It's almost empty. I'm sitting waiting for the next train with just one other person. He looks okay. A little odd, maybe. He is pacing. Guess he's running late. Looks maybe a little nervous.

Aaand, breathe. He is a totally normal person!

But maybe I should get on the train after his train. Just in case he has any kind of PLAN TO BLOW IT UP or anything. It's fine! I can wait.

"There is no terror in a bang, only in the anticipation of it."

❧ ALFRED HITCHCOCK ☙

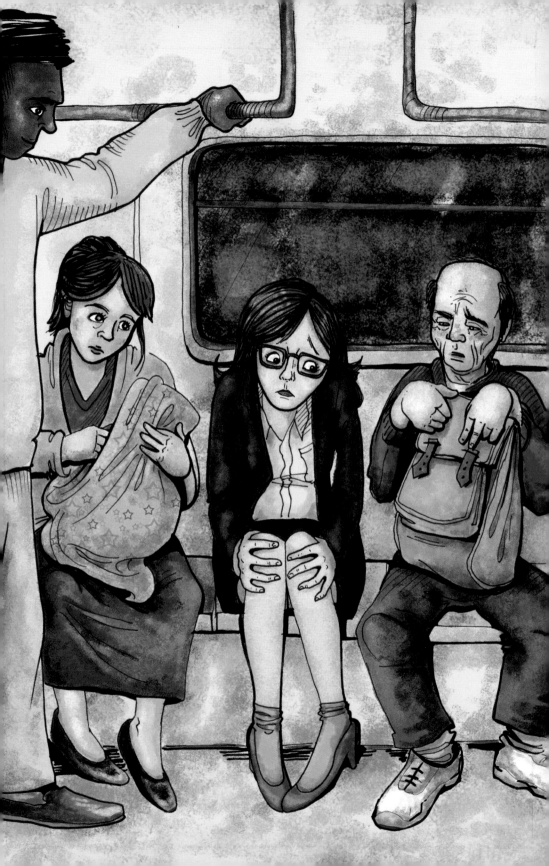

Women's magazines

Oh, why do they make me feel so BAD? I want to pick them up, I think it's a treat, I'm having a haircut, and I really think it'll be a good idea if I flip through a lovely glossy magazine. Half an hour later, I have a body image complex, a need to overspend, and have diagnosed myself with the latest disease that's "sweeping America."

Clothes first. Apparently I want a leopard-print peplum body-con velvet this-season's-must-have dress, $1000. I feel unfashionable and poor.

Celebrities next. Look how thin this one is! Look how fat that one is! Look how weary I am reading this!

And health. I now know, at least, that my fear of death stems mostly from these shrieking pages.

Being lumped into the "target audience" of these magazines makes me nervous . . . be it belonging to them or scared of not belonging!

"Who is it that can tell me who I am?"

ও WILLIAM SHAKESPEARE ৪৩

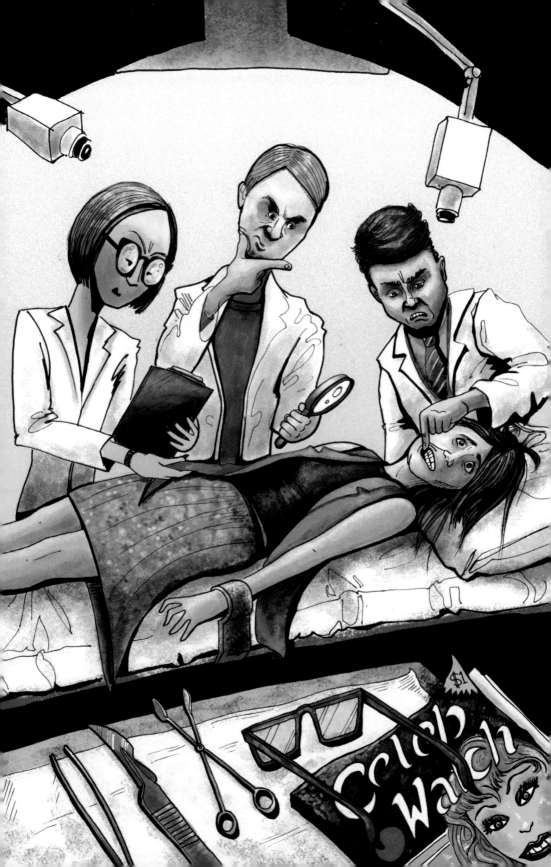

Having Children

I used to think that by the time I reached twenty-six, I'd have settled into a nice, stable relationship. So by the time I'm thirty, I'll be trying for a baby. Only I'm twenty-nine and single. And I feel a bit like a child still.

Claire told me she's never having children. Never, ever. Doesn't want them, never will. I'd love to be that brave! To actually make a decision about it! But instead, I cry at sad commercials that show kids all excited on Christmas morning and yet want to shout at the child screaming next to me when I'm trying to sit quietly and drink a coffee. Why doesn't any parent have anything nice to say about having children? They just look tired, depressed, and ill from their offspring's germs.

Those scary stories about fertility and how women are "waiting too long" are just written to scare vulnerable, terrified people like me. Right?

I have a long time before I need to start worrying.

Is fifty okay? I might have grown up by then.

"My mother had a good deal of trouble with me,
but I think she enjoyed it."

CR MARK TWAIN ᘐ

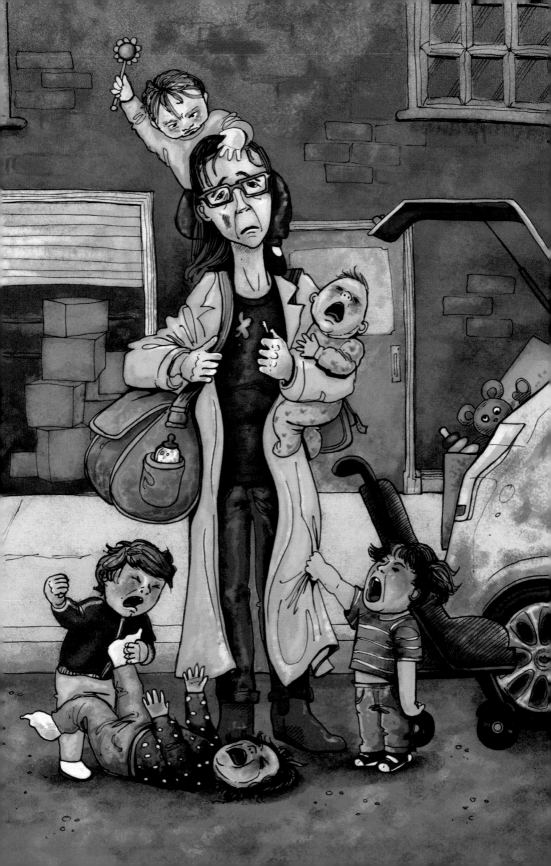

Bad Smells

I don't like inviting people into my home. A cat lives here, there is a damp area in the corner of the living room, and the bathroom is full of wet towels. I've been here all day. I don't know how it smells.

I'm going to a party tonight, which makes me anxious. At these kinds of events, people stand so close! At the last party I went to, the guy I was talking to had breath that meant I couldn't inhale for half an hour. It makes you wonder how bad your own breath is. For all I know, I am the stinkiest person anyone has ever met, but people havn't told me! The day I forget deodorant in my bag will be a frightening day. Today I realized I'd had fourteen sticks of gum in three hours. And this is all in the pursuit of good breath. Unfortunately, it hurts my jaw.

So, off to the party. Holding a bulging clutch bag with nothing that would fit inside it but a supersized extra-strength deodorant stick and a tub—a *tub*—of mints. It's all I had! Who needs a purse?

"We probably wouldn't worry about what people think of us if we could know how seldom they do."

CR OLIN MILLER EO

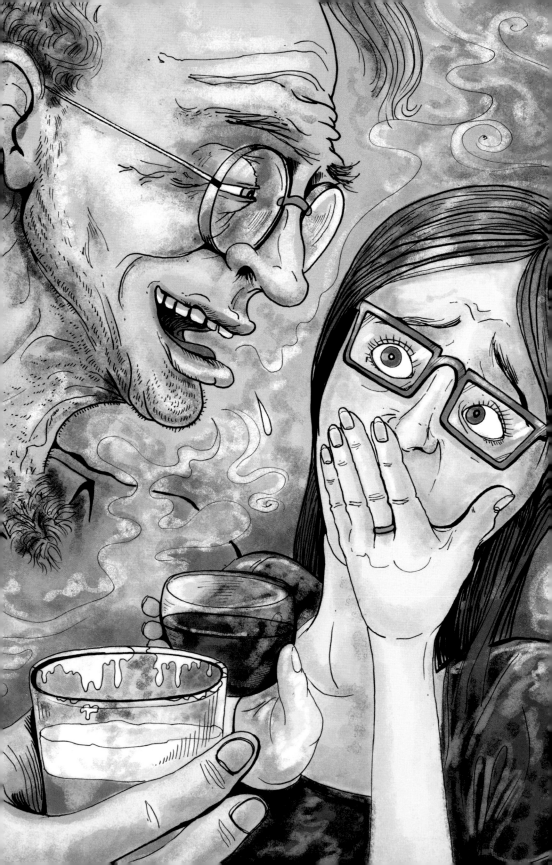

Finding "The One"

When I was fifteen, I went out with someone whose idea of a date was to practice playing the guitar for two hours in front of me, saying nothing. A lot of my dates since then have been similar. Somehow, I seem to go out with people whose "interests" take over their lives so much that they want me to be their cheerleader. I can't imagine doing the same thing. "Hey! I love drawing. I thought for our first date you could sit there while I draw this landscape and maybe you could make me tea every hour or so?"

When I was nineteen, I was with a stoner who played computer games as I sat and watched. This would go on every weekend until I went away to college, where I met some guys who had "just discovered" pot. Red eyes seemed to be everywhere. Munchies were relentless.

So, now I am sitting here eating dinner alone after Claire calls to tell me we should go on a double date with some colleagues of hers. Feeling a bit anxious about the idea. Will probably say no. If you want to avoid the mines, stay away from the minefield.

Time for an unrealistic romantic comedy and a bottle of wine.

"For me there's a daffodil in every dustbin."

ᏚᏒ Eric Sykes ℬ

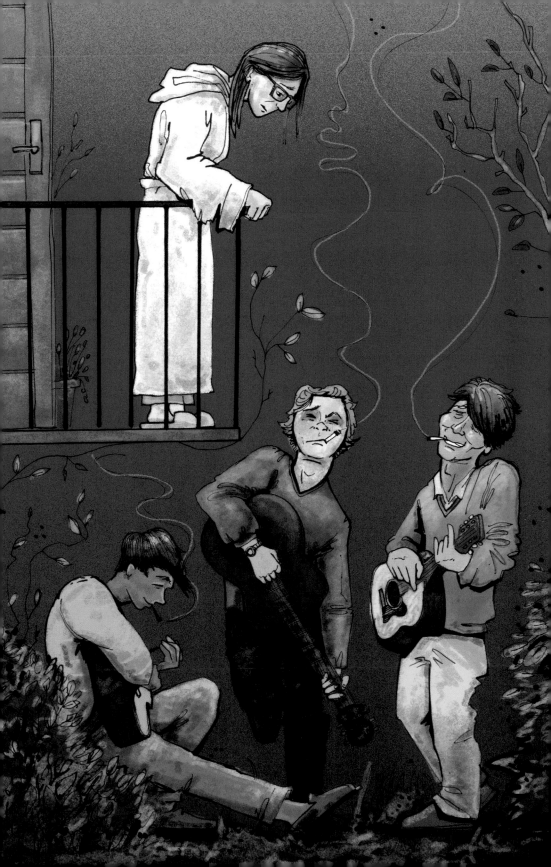

Exercise

Went for a run this morning. My knees and hips feel like they need immediate replacement. I might as well have been running in stilettos. But I read yesterday that you need to do thirty minutes of exercise per day. And that's just normal—you know, to avoid an early grave. What if you want to be all toned and beautiful? I think for me that would work out at around nine hours per day.

Some days are a recipe for anxiety. Like today. Half an hour at lunch looking at all the glossy magazines at the dentists, twenty minutes in a meeting with an impossibly fit colleague, all afternoon listening to people in the office talking about their PBs in the gym. There's a guy in IT who doesn't ever seem to get up from his chair; I found myself loitering around his desk a lot today to feel better. I even considered asking him on a date, until I saw him cough into his hand and wipe it on his pants.

Talking about exercise makes me tired. Pizza for dinner.

"Movement is a medicine for creating change in a person's physical, emotional, and mental states."

ᲪᲚ CAROL WELCH ᏠᎧ

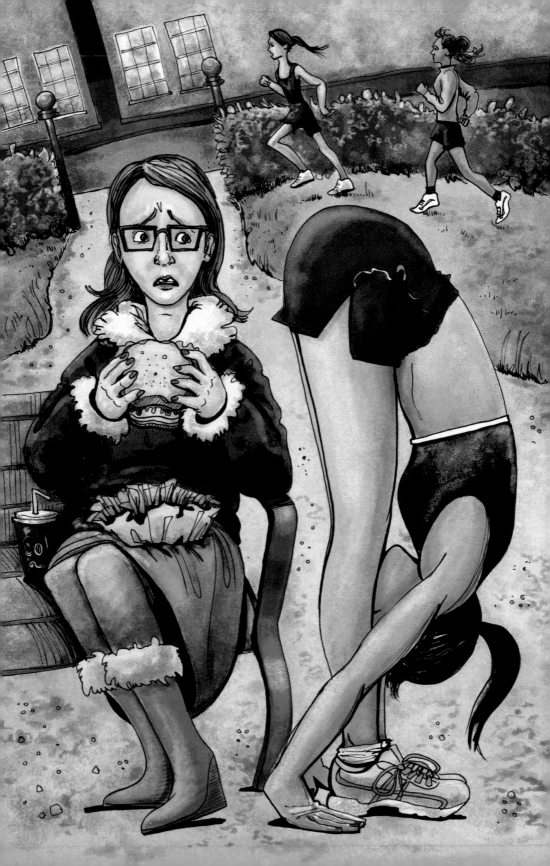

Hidden Ingredients

Had a headache-inducing trip to the grocery store. What is a stabilizer? Any food that contains something with the word "gum" in it can't be good, can it? What are all these e-numbers anyway?

"Diet" cola. Flavoring instead of sugar? Flavoring that turns into sugar?

I was so lost in imagining an evil professor cramming asbestos, tar, and roadkill into tiny jars that I didn't notice an old lady next to me. She'd been trying to reach something right above me for about ten minutes. "Excuse me," a man said and passed her a can. He looked at me like I'd run over his mother.

I ended up buying raw vegetables. My weekly shopping consisted of fourteen different kinds of vegetables and a bag of rice.

I got home, and I'm now going out again to buy potato chips, candy, and wine. I can't live like this.

*"Take care to get what you like
or you will be forced to like what you get."*

CR GEORGE BERNARD SHAW ᏸ

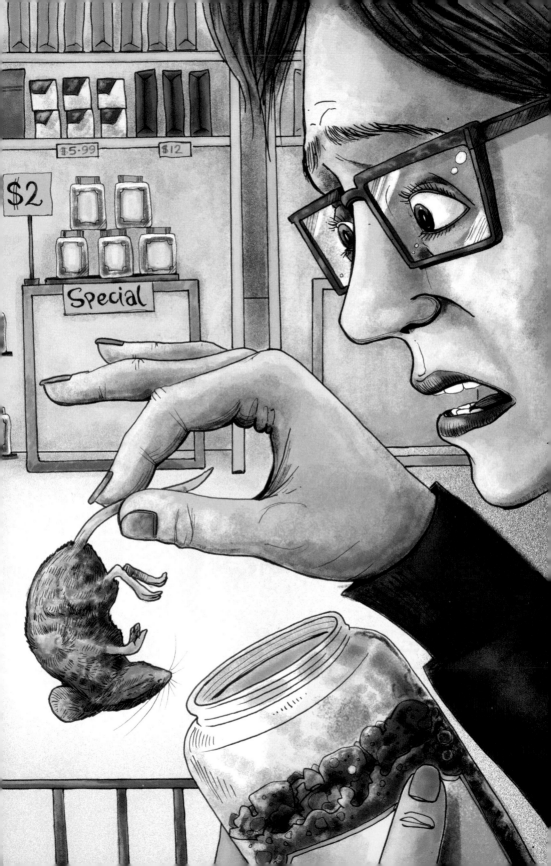

Forgetting Birthdays

I'm feeling sick. All day I have felt shaky and unwell. It's been three days since Claire's birthday, and I remembered in bed last night. She turned thirty-one without even a text from her best friend. I think she's now holding auditions for a new best friend. I immediately ran out before work this morning and bought her a Coen Brothers box set, left it on her porch with a note, and realized at work she already had it. We even watched Fargo from that exact set last week. Am I the stupidest person alive?

I feel really sick now, just left her three messages like a mad ex, and no reply. Why do I not write birthdays down on calendars? Why don't I set alarms all around the house telling me these things?

It's now midnight, and I'm mourning an incredible friendship. This is it, no more advice, no more support. I am alone.

2:00 a.m. Sent her an email for her to see at work telling her I can't be without her friendship. Got an automatic reply. "I am out of the office on vacation until next Monday and will be unable to receive calls and emails until then. I shall respond to your . . ." I remember her showing me the brochures now.

I am an idiot.

"Apology is a lovely perfume; it can transform the clumsiest moment into a gracious gift."

CR MARGARET LEE RUNBECK ଓ

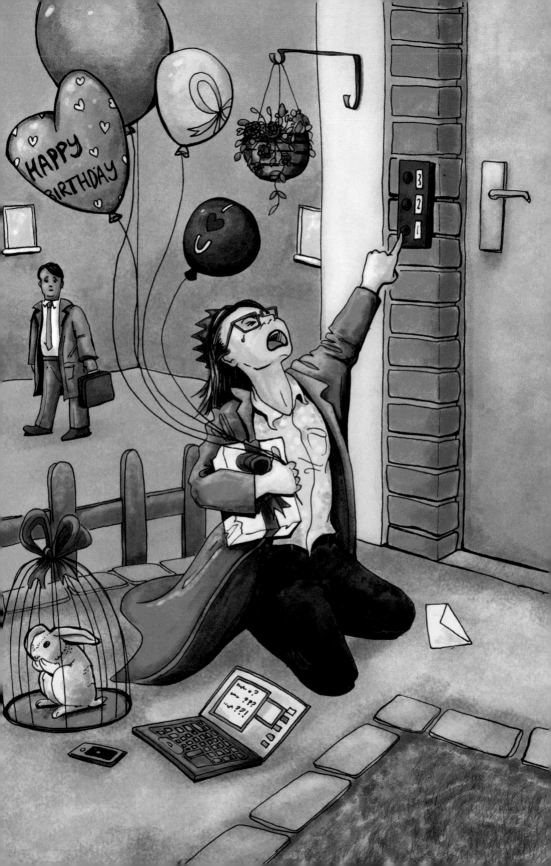

Murderers

Why is it that I see a man out for a walk alone and I assume he is going to kill me?

Every time I find myself in a beautiful, breathtaking part of the countryside, I imagine a dog walker finding my decomposing body weeks after a brutal stabbing.

I think of how I'd respond to a strange man coming toward me. My favorite scenario is to out-strange him. If I start singing "Memories" at the top of my lungs, while pirouetting, he might be more scared of me and walk away.

Quite often, I walk with my keys interlacing my fingers in my pocket, for a quick "Ha! Key-stabby-face!" maneuver should the need arise. He will reel backward and I shall make my getaway.

Sometimes I see a group of scary looking ten-year-olds farther down the road, so I stop, look at my phone, pretend to suddenly realize I have an urgent matter to attend to, and walk quickly in the other direction. Avoidance is key.

"Panic at the thought of doing a thing is a challenge to do it."

∞ HENRY S. HASKINS ∞

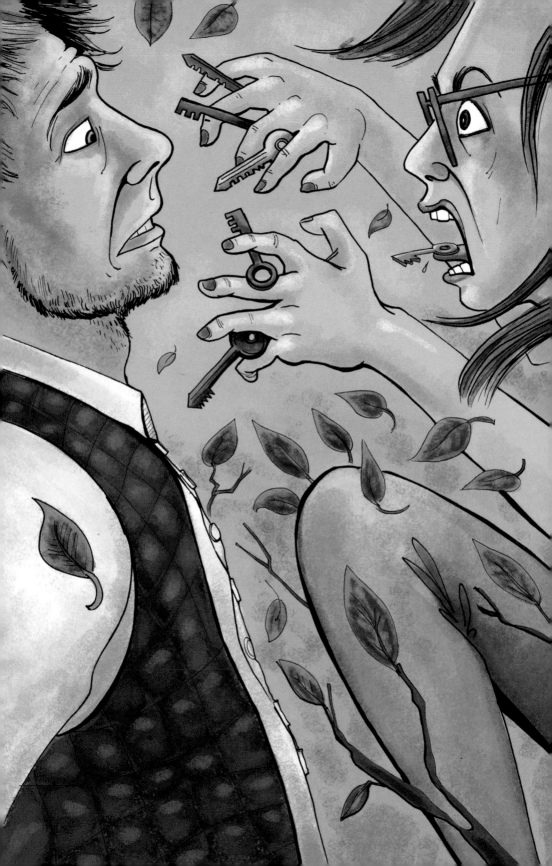

Small Talk

Claire is dragging me to some work function tonight. I am her "plus one." She told me there'd be some people from the art world I might want to talk to. She's an accountant. Hmm.

Still, there's a small chance I might need to impress someone, so my chest is feeling a little tight and I've checked to see if I still have my umbrella in my bag five times.

Claire says I need to master small talk. Sidling up to someone and remarking on a universal truth that will warm them to me. Easy. I have written a list of key words to mention on my palm: "Obama"; "Career crossroads"; "Religion"; "Anxiety"; and "Leonardo DiCaprio."

I just remembered Claire meant that I must avoid these subjects. God, what do I talk about?

"Talk to people about themselves and they will listen for hours."

ॐ Benjamin Disraeli ॐ

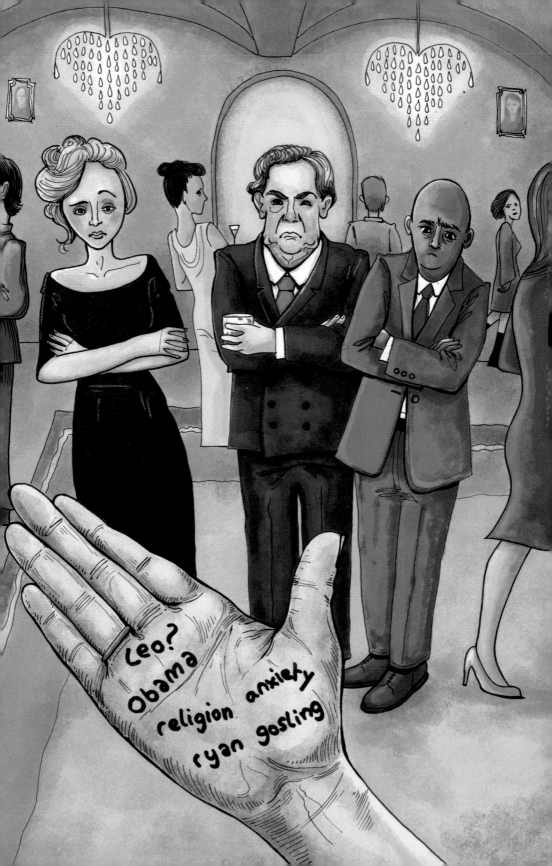

Getting Married

Confession: I don't want to get married. Did I ever want to get married? I think I just assumed I wanted to until I realized there was some kind of emotion that had to be involved. But people don't understand this. They just look at me and feel sorry.

As someone with a few ... a lot of ... anxiety issues, having a hundred people stare at me while I try not to spill things onto a white dress is not going to be the best day of my life. What if I fall onto an uncle walking down the aisle? What if everyone gets the wrong day? Organizing getting out of the house is difficult enough, let alone a year planning a wedding.

I know. I don't have a boyfriend let alone a fiancé. But it doesn't stop me from worrying about this pressure people put on me to find a "life partner." Everyone talks about weddings like I have to be excited. People look at me with so much pity when they talk about their "big day."

The pity gives me a headache.

"Regina," said Claire. "Screw them. You and I are going to be alone forever. Let's embrace it!" Not the pep talk I had in mind.

> *"Marriage is a great institution,*
> *but I'm not ready for an institution."*
>
> ❦ MAE WEST ❧

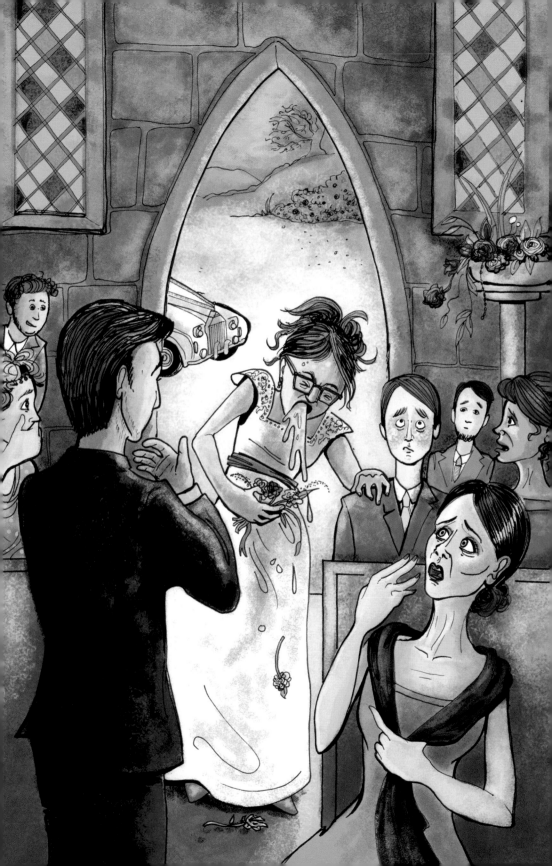

Drinking

How many liters of alcohol can I have per week again?

If there's one thing that makes me feel guiltier than anything, it's drinking. Even if I have one glass, I feel guilty the next day. My first thought when I wake up is, "So, your willpower failed again, Regina."

It's just . . . if there were only beer or spirits in the world, I might be okay. But while wine exists, how am I supposed to ignore it?

The best plan, I have realized, is to buy horrible tasting wine. I have half a glass and put it away. But that is a miserable existence.

Well, willpower, last night I had salad and water. The night before I had salmon stir fry and water. You can't ask any more of me if you want me to be happy. Tonight, I'm on the Malbec.

"Drink not the third glass."

ଔଷ GEORGE HERBERT ଔଷ

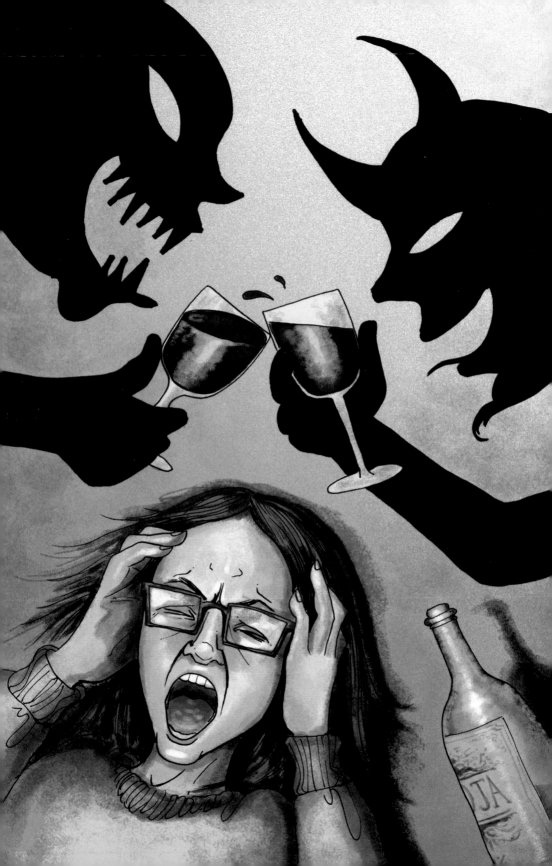

Time

Time is second only to Death as the source of all my fears.

I'm constantly doing depressing math in my head. The other day, I watched Sense and Sensibility. That film came out in 1995. Now those people are wrinkled. Then, they were smooth and plump and young. But 1995 wasn't all that long ago.

Friends finished in 2004. That's already a decade. I cannot go around doing normal things in my life knowing that Friends finished a decade ago.

And look at Brad Pitt. Look at him! He's gone from Golden Super Stud to Tired Chipmunk. Look at Johnny Depp! What has happened? How did I sleep through all that? Make it stop!

It has come to a stage where anything that wasn't filmed in the last six months makes me feel slightly unwell. Apart from one thing. I watch Friends at least once a week still and it is the greatest source of comfort anyone can self-medicate with. Ever. I can watch that and stop time and get back into my own head and everything is okay.

Everything is okay.

"The distinction between past, present, and future is only an illusion, however persistent."

ALBERT EINSTEIN

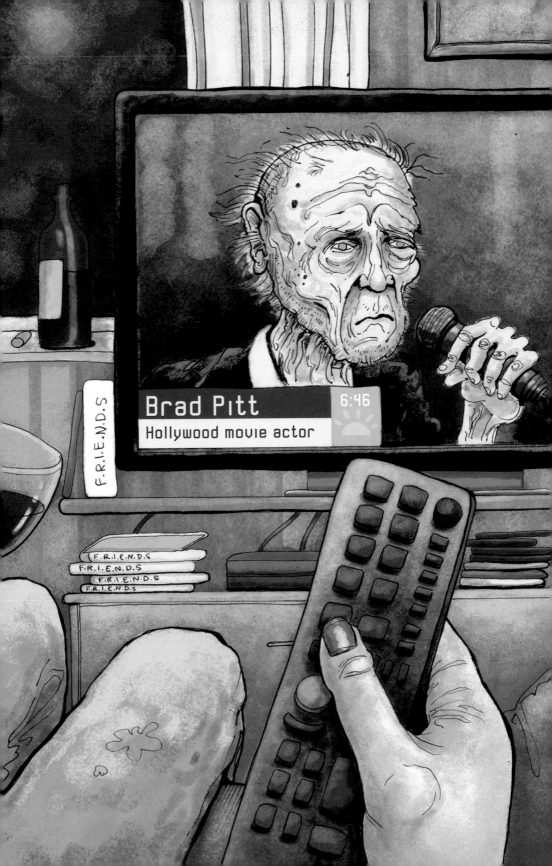

Jealousy

There are people you can feel happy for, but others bring with them an uncertain feeling in the pit of your stomach in terms of their successes. Yesterday, Claire and I were having coffee, talking about my lactose intolerance. I think Claire may have been slightly bored, as she was looking at her phone a lot. Then she yelled at me, "Regina! Look who's landed a presenting job on TV! Polly Kershaw! I know, right?"

Polly wasn't my most beloved acquaintance. She was always "behind the scenes" during a relationship I had at college, and when we broke up, she and my ex immediately started going out. I should have been okay with it but instead I danced around my apartment shouting "I KNEW IT!" and gulping down liters of wine.

So now I get to see her on TV! I can't help it. I feel a bit sick about it. I feel a bit jealous. Claire told me to eat another muffin and forget it.

But I might just go home and Google her and see how well she's doing . . . just to see . . .

"Jealousy is no more than feeling alone against smiling enemies."

ᏣᏛ Elizabeth Bowen ᏋᏗ

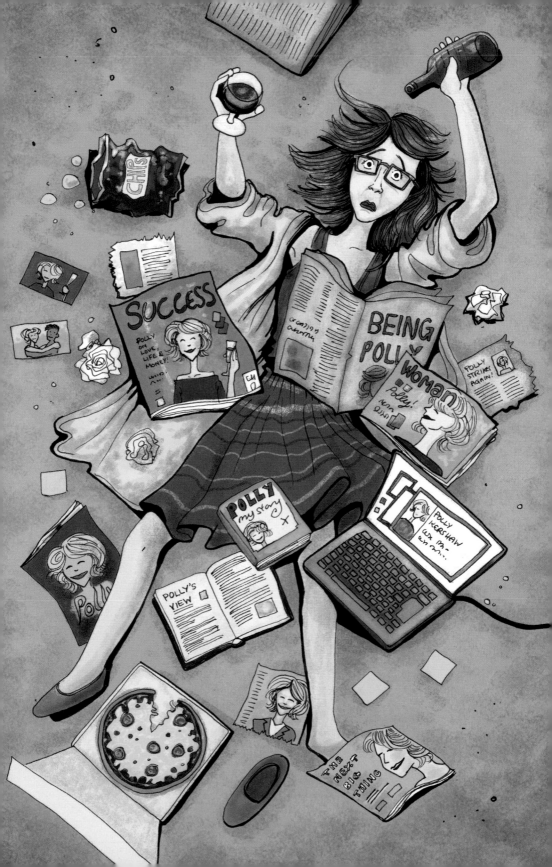

Driving

On my very first driving lesson, I was learning how to actually move the car when I saw a man standing on the sidewalk looking at me, laughing. Just standing there, laughing at me. I drove past him awkwardly, and I've never forgotten his face. I vowed I'd be a great driver and would prove all those sexist idiots wrong.

So my anger stems from the fact that I passed after my sixth attempt and driving makes me about as confident as I would be competing in the Super Bowl. Every time my test came, I'd start shaking, my foot would slip off the pedal, and I'd stall the car in the middle of the road.

I had to drive into town today to mail a package and, for about twenty-four hours before I had to do it, I was thinking about crashing, stalling, running out of gas, breaking down, and getting lost.

What happened? Nothing. It was okay.

Sauvignon Blanc.

"Face what you think you believe and you will be surprised."

WILLIAM HALE WHITE

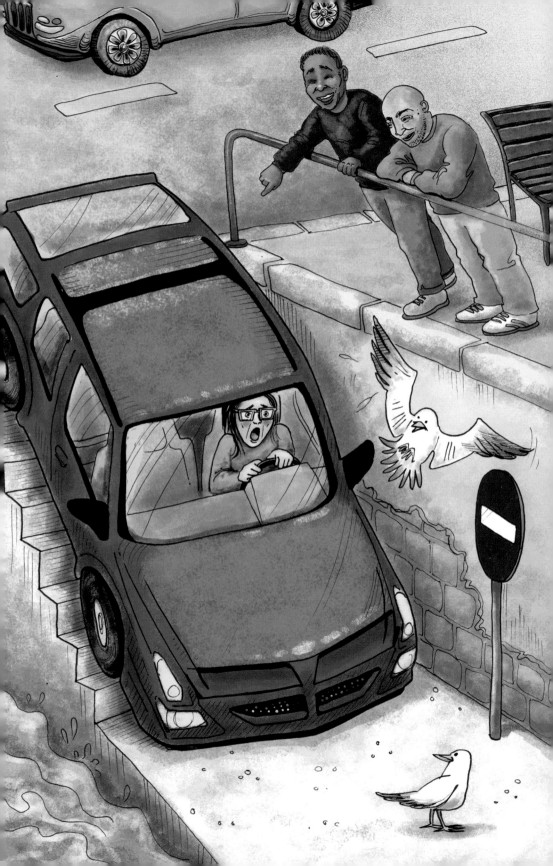

Celebrities

Claire has never been one to worry about how celebrities look or what they're saying. I try not to. But in my worst moments, I look down at myself and then look over at a picture of Olivia Palermo and feel like a screwed up paper bag.

I wonder how it is that no one in the public eye has toothpaste stains on them. Or breaks a heel or accidentally spits. I know. The paparazzi take some pretty unflattering shots, but those aren't the pictures I look at. I am sane enough not to buy those kinds of magazines. Just the glossy ones that contain impossibly perfect images of sparkly beautiful people . . .

Claire once said to me, "They're all just sacks of blood and guts like you and me, you know." I like to think that. I like to imagine them all squelching down the road.

"Celebrity is a mask that eats into the face."
CR John Updike EO

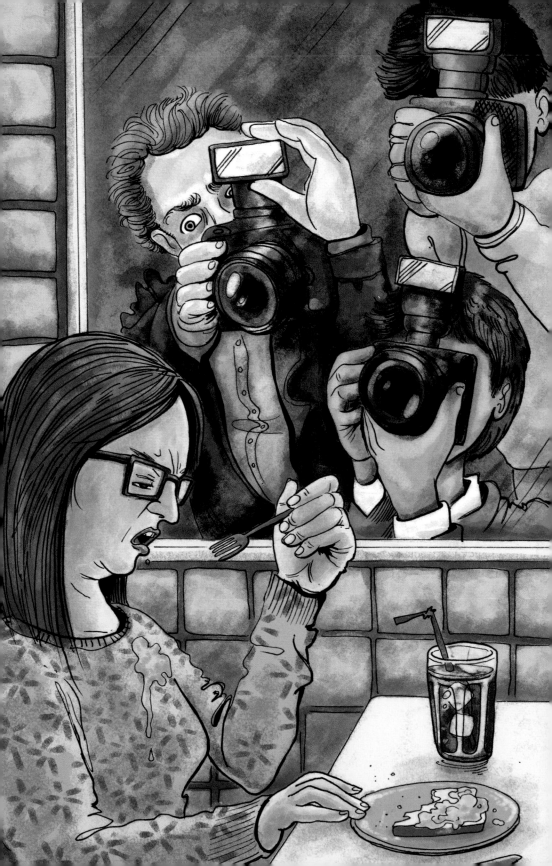

Internet Trolls

You can tweet "I like cake" and someone, somewhere, will get angry. Writing anything on the Internet for me isn't like it is for fifteen-year-olds. They write the most disgusting things on there and feel pretty good about themselves. "Ha, you look fat." "Go and kill yourself." Gotta love those teens. I spend most days wondering what I can say that won't incur the wrath of a band of shouters. I deleted a tweet for being too self-effacing. Then another for sounding arrogant. Then I wrote about something I was doing, which I deleted, as it sounded like I was showing off. So I mentioned I had bought some car cleaning products instead and deleted it for being the most boring thing I'd ever written.

Today I thought it was best to write nice, cultural things. "Interesting article about this new exhibition," I tweeted, smugly. "Watched a rather excellent new independent film last night," I said, feeling braver. "But I don't think much of the star—her performance was a bit wooden." Ah.

"Dick," someone tweeted. Obviously a fan of the actress.

"Braindead comment from @reginasmythe who obviously knows nothing about acting," wrote another.

"You're just an ugly loser," tweeted a third, helpfully.

Well, thanks for your input everyone. Lovely. I'm going to put the phone down, crawl under my comforter, and eat some potato chips. With a glass of Beaujolais.

"If you are not criticized, you may not be doing much."

CR DONALD RUMSFELD ꙮ

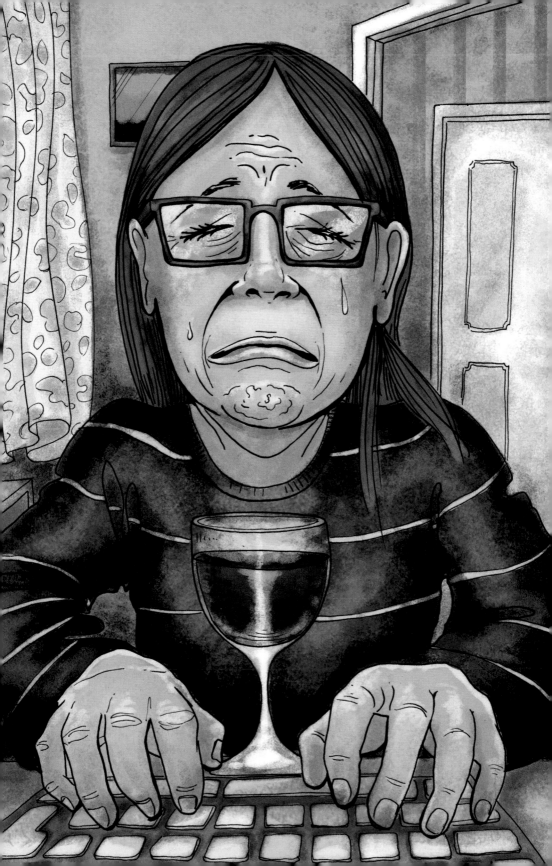

Sex

I've always been scared of sex for the first time with anyone. I thought I'd overcome that fear two weeks ago—initially, at least.

It involved going to a club with Claire and bumping into an "old friend." By that I mean someone I used a stare at a lot at work before he left.

So we got talking, and Claire kept deliberately leaving us alone, winking at me unsubtly. Before I knew it, it was the end of the night and I was inviting him up to my messy apartment. Drunkenness was the only reason for my bravery, but I still felt like it was my sixth driving test. I kept thinking I needed to move around like some kind of snake, effortlessly shedding my clothing and slinking into his grasp. But he was an old pro, and I was a clumsy lunatic.

I managed to throw my bag onto a lamp and smash it before seductively hiccupping in his face. He caressed my hair and I spent a good ten minutes undoing his belt. I used the belt to "lasso" him over onto the sofa, before falling onto it, forcing my knee firmly between the legs of his pants.

Am I ever going to feel confident in bed? Well, not with this guy. He left after I'd given him some frozen peas.

"Sex: the thing that takes up the least amount of time and causes the most amount of trouble."

CR JOHN BARRYMORE 80

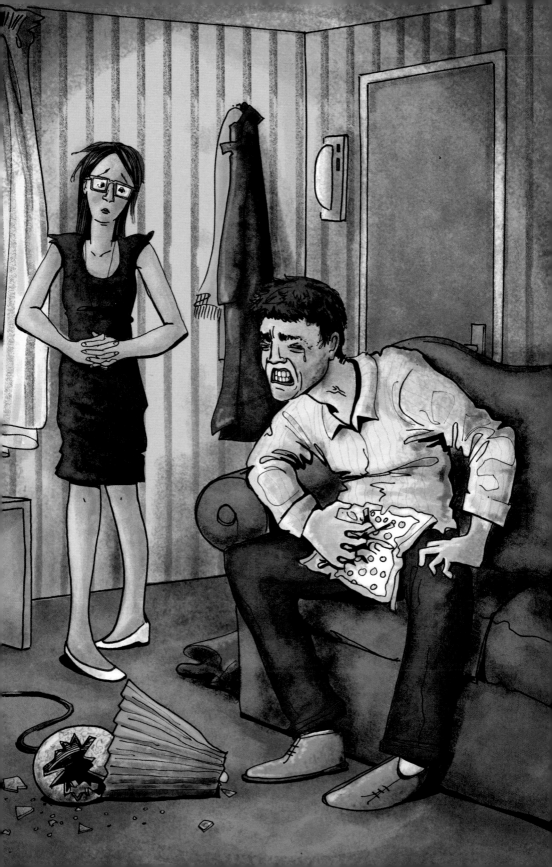

Family

"Regina, why don't you dress a little more *feminine?*" Mom pleaded when we were at the mall after work today. She had insisted on treating me, but the skinny jeans I was trying on weren't quite what she had in mind. She was holding up all these bright colors that clashed with my pallid skin tone. "I don't know why you like to look so drab all the time."

Over coffee, with fuchsia dresses and five-inch heels scattered all around us, I asked Mom if I could take her up on her offer to move back home. "Honey, absolutely. In fact, your father and I have already gone ahead and decorated your room. We knew this career of yours wasn't really taking off—I mean, it was only a matter of time before you came to your senses. I always said you should have pursued a more practical career, but you just wouldn't listen to me . . ."

After that inspiring chat, I decided to go and buy a pack of six chocolate muffins and watch three episodes of Friends in a row. I'm getting these frown lines . . .

My dad just called. "I hear you're coming home! That's great, chicken. We just need to work on your drinking and your job and you'll be right as rain. I have this fabulous jigsaw puzzle you can help me with in the evenings! Distraction is key, Regina. Distraction."

"Call it a clan, call it a network, call it a tribe, call it a family. Whatever you call it, whoever you are, you need one."

ʘ JANE HOWARD ʘ

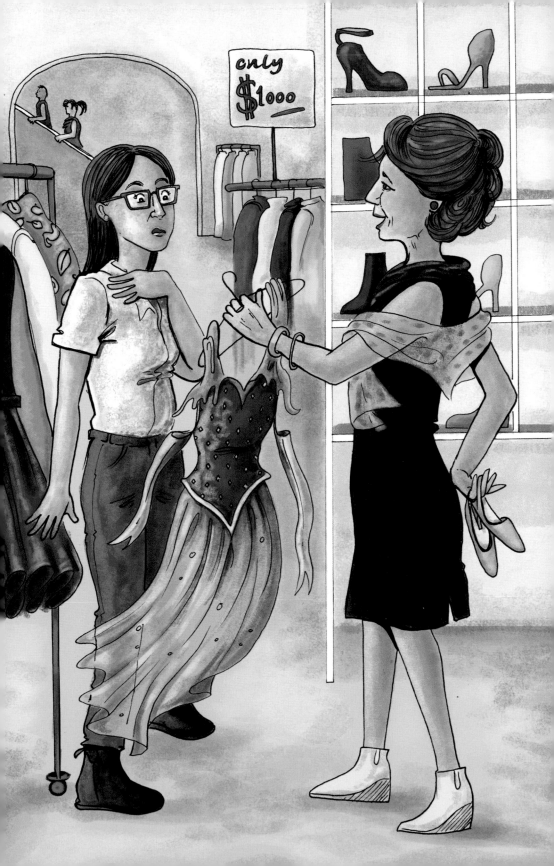

My Job

My job has been a source of much anxiety to me since I started there two years ago. On my first day, I walked in and felt sick, and things haven't changed much.

I'm paid pretty much the lowest amount you can get away with, and I try and keep myself to myself. We work in an open plan office, so even getting up is a real trial. Rising from my seat is an invitation for people to look at me. If the phone rings, I hate it. People listening to my wobbly voice talking to a client? It's enough to give me acid reflux. Once I answered the phone with a "thank you!" instead of a "hello." About five people laughed at me, and I was red for the entire day.

Then there's the kitchen. I can barely boil a kettle of water without getting in the way of one of my bosses, shaking sugar all over them or inappropriately touching them by accident. All work kitchens should be BIG, okay? A small kitchen for thirty people is just not practical!

There is only one place that is my sanctuary. The ladies' room. I just have to make sure I don't stay there too long, as I believe my boss already thinks I have bowel problems. She is right, though.

"Far and away the best prize that life offers is the chance to work hard at work worth doing."

CR THEODORE ROOSEVELT ЯƆ

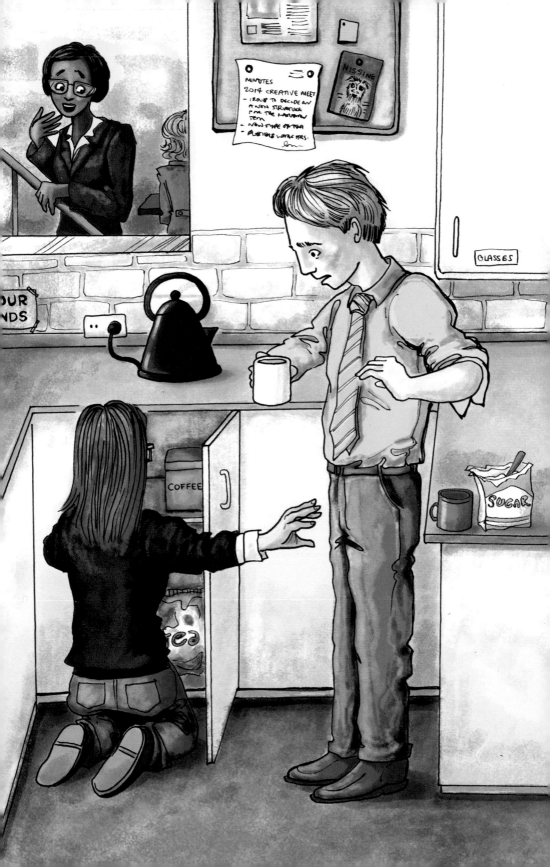

My Car

With every mile I drive, there's an expectation that I will have an issue with my car. I drove to work today and had to smile nervously at a pedestrian on the sidewalk as I attempted to restart my car at the lights. This middle-aged man was just standing watching me as I tried four times to get Brenda started again.

Brenda is my Pontiac Aztec. She's never won any beauty pageants, she drives like she has a cold, but she's all I have, and I'm not in a position to upgrade. I've been to three interviews in this car, and I have the distinct impression she lost me two of those jobs.

The thing that really makes me anxious, though, is this vision I have where I'm driving home in the dark from somewhere isolated, without a charged phone, and Brenda dies on me. I've dreamed about this scenario every few weeks. It sometimes involves a murderer waiting in the bushes for such an opportunity, sometimes not. This depends on the kind of day I've had.

I can't exactly blend in, either. Brenda is a bright burnt orange color, with that kind of metallic sheen reserved for attention seekers. Fabulous.

"You were born an original. Don't die a copy."

ℭℜ JOHN MASON ℬ℧

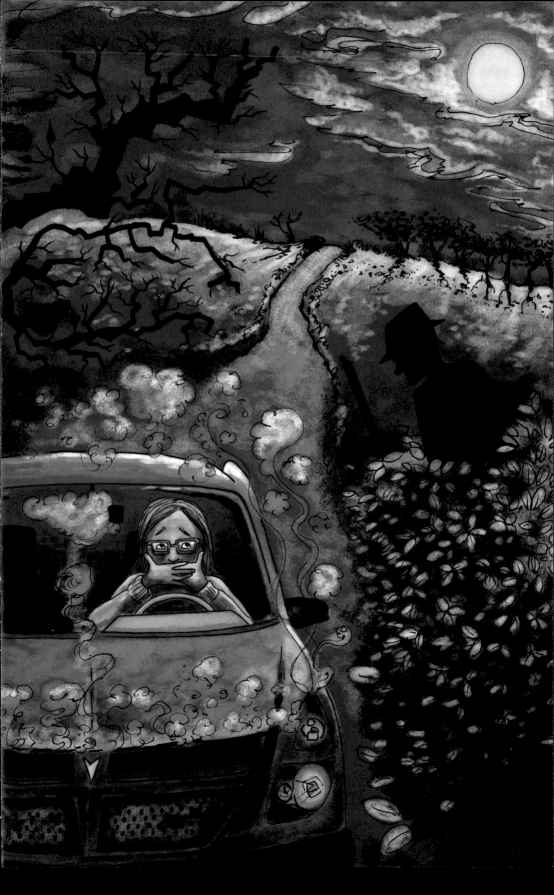

Senility

I always thought you had to wait until you were a little older to walk into a room and forget why. But this is my reality: I'm constantly gazing into the middle distance, walking past places I need to go, missing turns, standing in doorways as if waking from a sleepwalking episode. This worries me a lot. Is my brain winding down already?

"Regina, you just put ketchup on that muffin. Are you okay?" Claire said earlier, all too used to my behavior.

"Claire, I think I'm losing it."

"You're not, Regina. You are just so caught up in your anxieties that you can't see what's in front of you."

I'm not convinced by this. Sometimes I go to bed at night and my thoughts seem to swirl around. I lose grip on what I'd thought about moments before, and I flail around trying to regain normal thought. It's like a hand is forcing my head into deep water, before forcing it upward again.

So, there you have it. I'm losing my mind. My brain has aged at a rate of five times the normal amount. By next week, I'll have forgotten Claire's name and I'll be shouting at her for coming too close.

"Everyone is more or less mad on one point."

CR RUDYARD KIPLING ☙

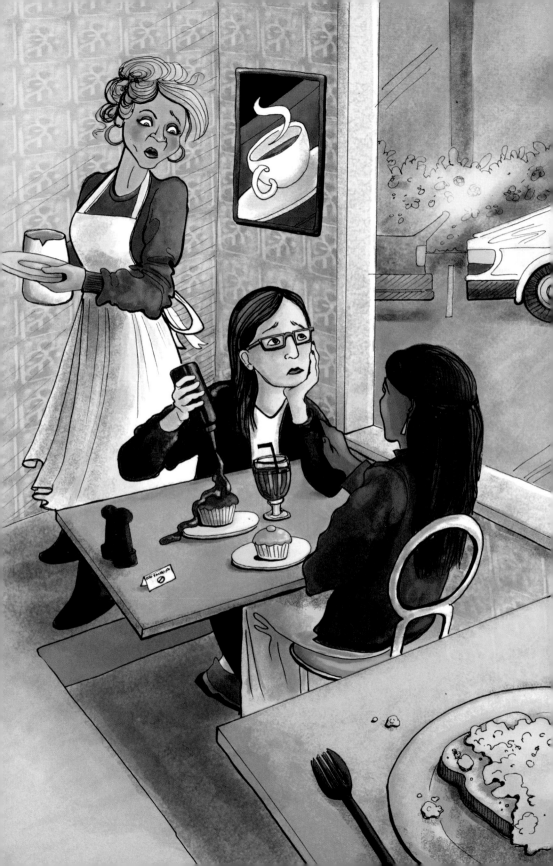

Theft

This morning was a typical morning. I walked around the apartment, closing windows and locking doors, before grabbing my keys and making for the door. I then turned and did another circuit to check all those windows I had previously checked.

I then left the building, walked down the street, and started fixating upon the cat door. Someone could reach through that and unlock the door if they had very long arms. The length of this criminal's arms wouldn't leave my thoughts, so I marched back home to block up the hole. Noticing a necklace I had left in the hallway, I scolded myself for flagrantly inviting thieves to smash through a window and take it.

By the time I'd finished "securing" my home, I was half an hour late for work.

I think a lot about how easy it would be for someone to steal from me. When someone calls me at night and my phone lights up like a lantern, I try to answer it inside my coat. I hug my purse in bars and restaurants tightly. I'll be sitting in a nice restaurant and will have my purse on my lap underneath my napkin.

And watch out, all you loiterers. If any of you hang near me for too long, I'm calling the police.

"Considering how dangerous everything is nothing is really very frightening."

GERTRUDE STEIN

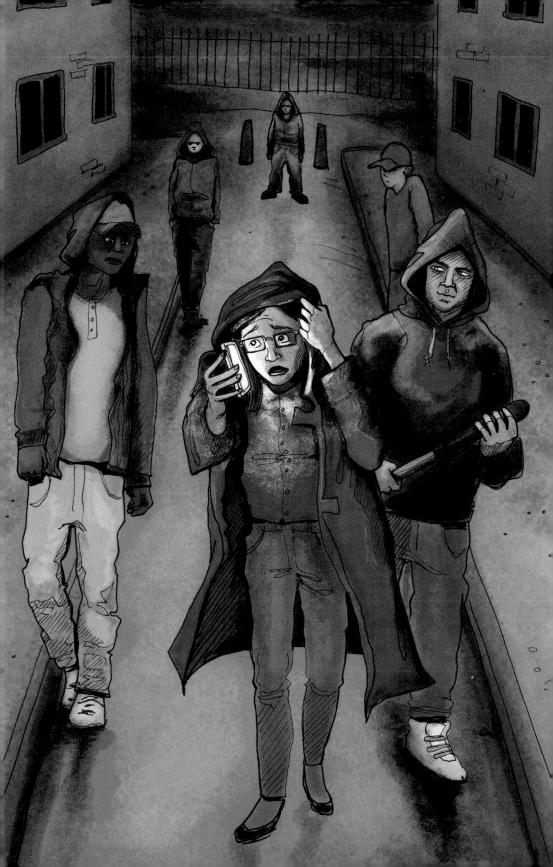

Hygiene

I'm not one of those people who scrubs herself obsessively every few minutes. I know I could easily evolve into doing that, but my concern is mainly other people's hygiene. Once you become aware of it, stomach-churning atrocities are suddenly all around you.

Today, I was on the subway and decided against sitting on the only available seat, due to a weird greenish liquid pooling in its center. Unfortunately, though, I had to stand near a man who ruined my morning. He was a young, well-dressed man on his way to work, briefcase in hand. He had his head down, and the cold he was suffering meant that his nose would run with his head at that angle. So he snorted; a huge, phlegm-soaked outburst, made a swallowing sound, and then exhaled extravagantly. I looked desperately around to see if anyone else had reacted each time, but there was not a flicker.

Suddenly you realize how disgusting humans are, and you anxiously try to avoid them. I don't like touching handrails. I avoid seats, poles, and loose change without gloves, and then scuttle home to wash my hands.

"Dirt is only matter out of place."

ᑫ᙭ JOHN CHIPMAN GRAY ᙭ᑫ

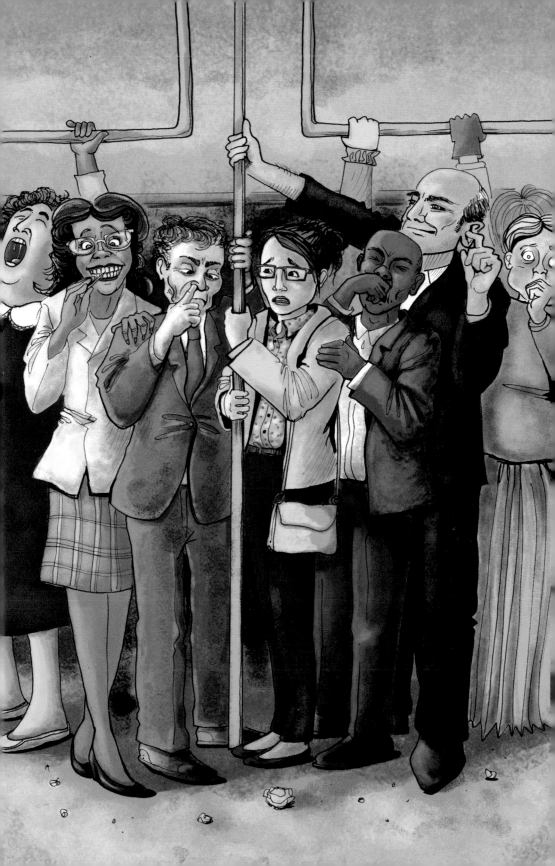

Nighttime

I woke up last night and thought about how broke I am. The covers were getting more and more heavy and hot, and the pillow was a deflated child's balloon, rubbing statically against my hair. My chest started to become heavy and tight, and my breathing got shallow. I tried to push the money issues from my mind, but then I imagined all the things I have to do this month: buy my mom a birthday present; pay the last lump of rent before I finally move out; meet some old work colleagues for a drink.

"Cancel the drinks," I thought. "Cancel that lunch I had planned with Claire. Cancel the order for new underwear. I can do without an umbrella. I can put up with the rain." I was about to cancel Mom's birthday when I think I must have fallen asleep.

Waking up an hour before the alarm this time, I started mentally compiling things I could sell. "Apart from my car, I have nothing! What do I do? What can I possibly do to save myself? I feel so sick . . ."

And then the alarm. I checked my phone and saw a text from Mom. "Can't wait for you to move back in," it said. "Just think of all the rent you'll save! You'll soon have enough saved up again."

I breathed. She is right. I can get through this. As long as I don't go to bed ever again.

"Fear can keep us up all night long,
but faith makes one fine pillow."

ᎧᏒ PHILIP GULLEY ᏖᎧ

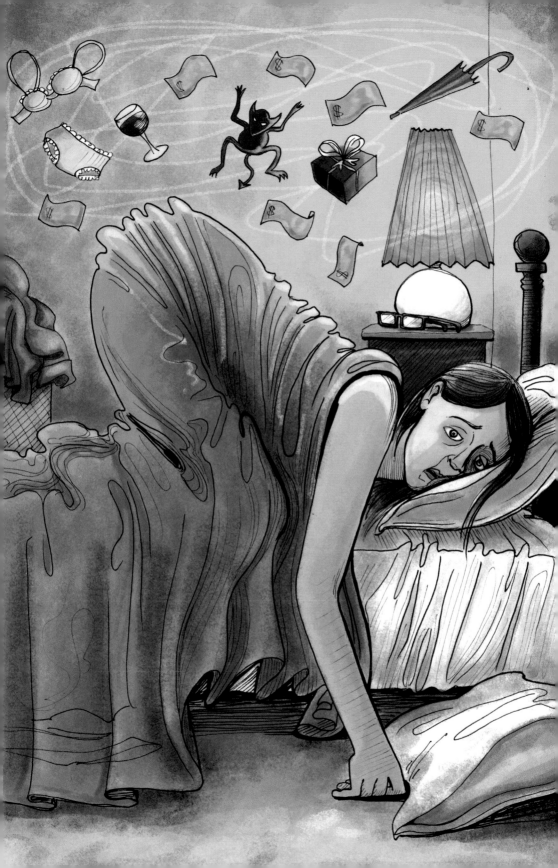

The Gym

I've been going to the gym for about two years. My anxiety tells me that if I stop going now, I will immediately double in size and start wheezing. So I go, and each time I have to put up with a thing I can only describe as "other people."

Last night, I was waiting for a weight bench to become free as a huge muscle-clad Adonis stretched out on one, talking to his friend lifting weights next to him. I tried my best to look hungrily at the bench, but he didn't notice and continued talking. His friend got up and started to dry himself off with his tiny towel, so I gave it a minute and scooted on over. "Excuse me," the friend said. "I'm using that." I looked at his physical form—caveman-like—slouching about two feet from the bench. I looked back at the bench. "Oh, okay. Sorry," I said, and walked away.

My confidence at the gym is always at an all-time low and not because of body confidence, but due to the fitness fanatics that surround me. I feel like they're looking at my "difficulty" level on my treadmill, smirking. They're probably watching to see if I cut corners. I feel SO. WATCHED.

Paranoia? Maybe. But I'm watching them, too.

"Do it, and then you will feel motivated to do it."

CR ZIG ZIGLAR ༡༠

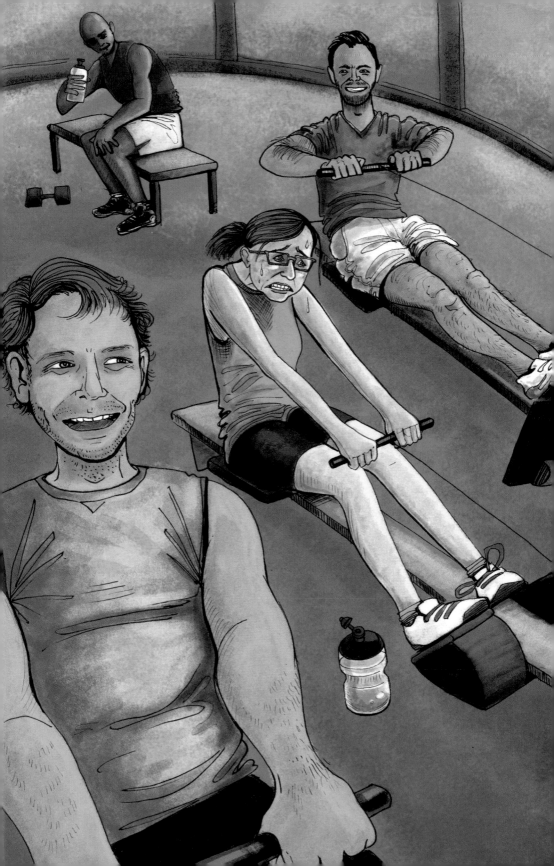

Enemies

Claire called me this afternoon to tell me that someone had written something horrible about me on her blog. "Don't get upset about it, Regina. It's just Hazel being her usual, awful self. Ignore her."

Hazel is my Allocated Enemy. Everyone has to have at least one, I have discovered. I used to work with her, and I got the promotion she wanted. I got to serve people cheese instead of stack shelves when we were both seventeen. Ever since then, she's wanted to get one up on me. I sometimes think her entire career has been built around being more successful than me.

"Just saw Regina Smythe looking like a middle-aged male librarian at a party. Get some style advice, Regina! LOL" is what Hazel wrote. I smiled as I read it, then disappeared home to stare at my wardrobe for three hours.

Is she right? Do I really look like an old man? She always gets to me. She always senses what I'm worrying about and goes for it. Last year it was her dating a guy I had a crush on. The moment they got engaged, she tweeted about how I had "lost out."

Next year it'll be her comments about me living at home again. "Poor, sad Regina. Let's all laugh at Regina. Isn't she pitiful?"

"Don't be distracted by criticism. Remember—the only taste of success some people have is when they take a bite out of you."

CR ZIG ZIGLAR 80

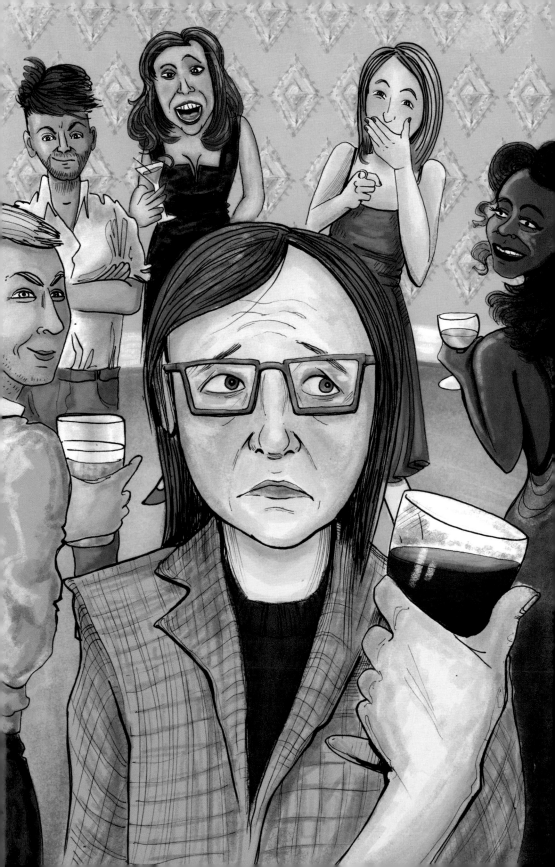

Loneliness

When I'm alone, I'm so aware of my head, and my thoughts, and sometimes these thoughts can overwhelm me. My anxieties can swoop in, and I feel like I'm trapped with them in a tiny box, unable to get out.

Last night I was packing up my things for the move, and I found some old photos. Forgotten people at college, a fancy dress party, a smiling tipsy Regina with her arms around her friends. It made me feel so alone. I thought of that time as a hundred years ago. It was like looking at photographs from a school textbook. I put the pictures away and pulled a blanket around my shoulders and cried.

That night was the loneliest I'd had in a long time. I felt like the room was shrinking. I stared at the ceiling and imagined being a confident, happy person again.

This morning Mom arrived in her old jeans and gray blouse to help me move. I could almost have called her drab. "Moving day!" she sang at me, as Dad followed her in.

So now I'm in my old room. We spent the evening watching old comedies, shared a huge pumpkin pie, and Dad squeezed my shoulders, saying, "This is a new start, Regina! A new beginning for you. It's all about how you view it."

Claire texted to see if I wanted to go out for a drink. "I think I'll pass," I replied. "Gotta start saving for this new start I've begun."

"Good! Now you need to think about the possibility of things actually going right for you. Won't that be a fun change?"

Very funny, Claire.

"No my friend, darkness is not everywhere,
for here and there I find faces illuminated from within; paper
lanterns among the dark trees."

CR CAROLE BORGES ⁊

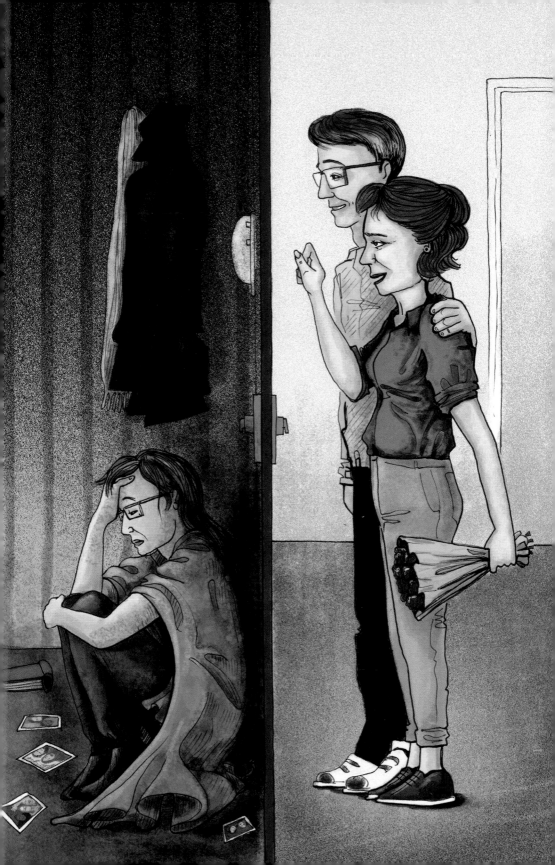

Skyhorse Publishing books may be purchased in bulk at special discounts for sales promotion, corporate gifts, fund-raising, or educational purposes. Special editions can also be created to specifications. For details, contact the Special Sales Department, Skyhorse Publishing, 307 West 36th Street, 11th Floor, New York, NY 10018 or info@skyhorsepublishing.com.

Skyhorse® and Skyhorse Publishing® are registered trademarks of Skyhorse Publishing, Inc.®, a Delaware corporation.

Visit our website at www.skyhorsepublishing.com.

10 9 8 7 6 5 4 3 2 1

Library of Congress Cataloging-in-Publication Data is available on file.

Cover design by Danielle Ceccolini
Cover illustration credit Bethany Straker

Print ISBN: 978-1-62914-460-3
Ebook ISBN: 978-1-63220-187-4

Printed in China